I0488865

Insider Tips on Transitioning to and Getting the Most Value Out of Your Healthcare Career

And Reaching Your Goals With Minimal Debt

by Jeffrey A. Gaines, R.N.

ISBN: 1500332747
ISBN 13: 9781500332747

Table of Contents

Introduction

Are you happy with your station in life? What would you do if you could turn back the clock? What would you change about yourself or your situation? Would you have more money? More time? More freedom? Of course, many of us would choose money. Money is the CREAM (cash rules everything around me) of life. And for one reason or another, we all find ourselves chasing it. Obviously, we have not discovered how to go back in time, which is why it is so important to make good decisions the first time around.

The United States is the greatest country in the world, but when it comes to debt, it can be unforgiving. Like many throughout my lifetime, I have made many good and bad decisions and have had to suffer the consequences. But we learn from our mistakes so that we won't repeat them. This is why it is so painful to see so many Americans put in situations where they are forced to make choices in the heat of the moment. The sudden economic downturn, the housing bubble, government shutdowns, and our own bad decisions have forced many people to reinvent themselves to survive. Currently, we have a new phenomenon pending known as the student loan bubble that is threatening to wreak havoc on many postgraduate degree recipients. Constant and ever-growing college tuition costs have forced many students to borrow astronomical amounts of money, not only to reach their educational goals, but to pull themselves up by their bootstraps and reach a better quality of life for themselves and their families. Thousands of those are finding themselves in a much worse situation than when they started, especially the teenagers who do not plan a way to pay back those loans after graduation. They may not have foreseen a struggle to find a job after they receive their degrees. Also, they did not have the foresight to research what jobs would be in demand. And even those who were able to find jobs are feeling overwhelmed by their monthly payments.

A college education is one of the few ways known to Americans to change their financial situation. Unfortunately, without a college degree, it is very difficult to make enough money, not just for the necessities of life, but to take care of your family and live above the poverty line. Those who made well-researched decisions about their future are the ones who are thriving and will continue to thrive in this economy. Those who have not have had to find ways—often creative ways—to utilize alternative methods in achieving their educational goals. Today, because of the high cost of education, it is not enough to educate yourself on what you think you're good at or what you think you might love to do. One must take a long, hard look at the job market and position oneself to take advantage of the occupations that are and will be in demand. High-profile careers that we were told as kids to reach for—doctors, lawyers, dentists, even anesthetists—are very costly because of the high tuition, and five, ten, fifteen years down the road these professionals are finding themselves unable to complete their studies or enjoying the fruits of their achievements until they pay off the balance of their debts. This unfairly demotes all of their hard-earned efforts and accomplishments to living within their worth and often below their means, leaving them to eke out a substandard living.

I am here to tell you that there is light at the end of the tunnel. There are pathways in achieving your desired education in which you do not have to end up in deep debt, and to the contrary, it can lead to financial freedom upon graduation. I'm here to tell you that not only can you maintain your debt freedom while studying for your degree, but you can enhance your ability to build wealth after you have found employment. Pathways exist that not only lead to upper-management positions but can lead to self-employment, as well as starting your own business. Although there are alternatives, they are not short-term remedies, and you must have patience and diligence and be willing to take the long road in order to resist the temptation of the short road toward long-term debt.

I'm a registered nurse. I have been working as a nurse since 1997, and I also hold a bachelor's degree in communication. I've held various positions in management, sales, and retail, but the majority of my career I have spent working as a nurse. I've had the opportunity to work in various specialties, such as research, gastroenterology, dialysis, IV, orthopedic, med-surg, and geriatrics. I've also worked as a travel nurse, contract nurse, and full-time, part-time, and per-diem PRN in large institutions such as local and state hospitals, as well as outpatient clinics. Working in almost every capacity in the nursing profession, I have learned the ins and outs of the industry and how it works.

During my tenure as a registered nurse, I have been privileged to learn many skills in various specialties that enhance the position I currently hold. A big part of the nurse's duties is to supervise and troubleshoot any situation to promote quality health care. I've also learned that in order to maintain a steady increase in your wages, you have to do one of two things: obtain a higher degree or hustle, as I refer to it. That may sound funny coming from a professional nurse, but those are the facts. Although nurses are paid a fairly decent wage for their services, the wage increases tend to be very small: on average, 2 percent per year, and those increases are with outstanding evaluations from management. In this text, I will talk about different ways to consistently increase your wages over time at a much higher rate than most corporations and institutions are willing to give nurses who stay in their positions for long periods. This rule of thumb is not only relegated to the nursing field but health care in general. Most nonmanagement employees punch a clock. In my opinion, punching a clock is much better than being salaried. Although your time is managed by a clock, you do have the opportunity to earn overtime. I have been given many opportunities to go into management positions, but in my opinion, the wage increase is not commensurate with the increased responsibilities; on the contrary, if your goal is to join management then by all means take advantage of the opportunity.

Attending nursing school is probably one of the best investments I've ever made. Of course, in 1997, community college was much cheaper than it is today. I graduated with no debt and paid under $10,000 for the whole two years. It was a grueling program, but I was intent on making it through. It was much harder than obtaining my bachelor's degree, which was under $25,000 for four years, including room and board. But because student loans were so easy to get, at graduation I still owed approximately $15,000 because of student refunds used for my personal benefits. Although that is a large sum, it is nothing compared to what the average college graduate in 2014 is contending with. And I can admit with much shame that my amount grew to almost $25,000 until I just recently paid it off in early 2014.

Unfortunately, like many today, my mind-set led me astray from the importance of quickly paying off my debts and maintaining a good credit score. Instead of taking advantage of the opportunity I made for myself by becoming a nurse and working diligently to save and invest, and because I had very few responsibilities other than myself for most of those years, I worked intermittently and took many days off to do what I wanted to do, my "honeymoon period." Unfortunately, many of those hours were unproductive, and just within the last ten years or so, I've come to realize how important it is to take advantage of being an in-demand professional, working hard in the initial part of your career so you have more freedom toward the end. I've owned numerous cars and homes, and I've spent a lot of money on frivolous goods and services. I've incurred many fees and penalties from various sources because I was lax in accepting the responsibilities of my deeds and debts. I accumulated a lot of "stuff," for which I had nothing to show. In all, I probably squandered over $100,000 during my career, which should be sitting in an interest-bearing mutual fund of my choosing. I point this out to inform you that it is never too late to pick yourself up by your bootstraps and begin again.

I learned a lot through trial and error and wasted a lot of time, and that is one of the biggest reasons why I'm writing this book. I'm hoping that I can save many of you time and money normally wasted learning lessons through trial and error. Just to give you some insight, I am forty-seven, paid cash for my house, have no car note, and totally debt free as of this writing. I'm looking forward to building wealth enough to be able to work voluntarily by the time I am fifty-nine. For those of you younger than I am, you must wake up and smell the coffee. Take advantage of the opportunities before you. Whether you're just starting out or in the midst of graduating, there is abundance for the employee and opportunities for those who want to be more than just employees. Follow the correct pathways I suggest in this book, and you will have the freedom to become whatever you want and live the lifestyle you deserve.

High Schoolers

Hopefully, this text will reach you before you decide to enter into an institution of higher education. If it does, my hope is that by this time in your life, you have been smart or lucky enough to have escaped the grips of the legal system. For many of the unlucky ones, it is a sad state of affairs. Once it has captured you, your choices become very limited. Not only do you become subservient to those who have large stakes and investments in its existence, but the laws within it are structured to keep you in bondage forever. You must not become entangled in its web. I understand that for many it is not a matter of choice; it is a way of life. But for those who have the chance to go in a different direction, you must lead the way for those who will come after you—your sons, daughters, and those seeds yet to be planted.

I have so many friends and relatives who consciously chose to make themselves victims of the system when they had the opportunities open to them to do the right things. Unfortunately, the lure of "the streets" and all that it entails led them on a course toward making negative decisions that would affect them for the rest of their lives. Make yourself aware of the consequences of your actions early in life. Think of all the things yet to be achieved through education. And be aware that one small infraction can lead to physical and/or mental imprisonment. Whether a felony, a misdemeanor, or a citation, become educated on the implications of each penalty. Each one carries with it the stain of indignation, whether it was righteously given or not. I consider myself lucky because, growing up where I did, there was plenty of opportunity to get into trouble. I did not always make good decisions; I was just lucky enough not to have gotten caught. As I look back, I was no better than the friends and relatives mentioned earlier, except I didn't take measures as far or get in "too deep," as some would say. Because of my personality, or possibly my fear of the streets, I focused more on sports and did not become engulfed in the wave of illicit activity that a lot of my friends were engaged in. I was lucky, and if those unlucky ones who got caught had not gotten caught, they could have easily achieved the same goals I have. Don't be one of the unlucky ones.

Stay at home for as long as possible. Food, clothing, and shelter are the staples of life. Wherever you go, you cannot survive without them. And if you leave home, you will have to pay for them. I know you've been in this place for sixteen, seventeen, eighteen years, dealing with your mom, dad, sisters, and brothers, and you are ready to go. In 2014, even as a teenager, you must take into consideration the costs of your decisions. There are so many graduates who wished they had saved the money they spent on dorm rooms and apartments and put it toward their tuition. Yes, it's a lot of fun to live on your own at that age, but in order to reach your goals debt free in this day and age (unless you have the finances to easily afford that type of lifestyle), you are better off living at home. Not only is the shelter that you'll need draining your finances, but all the other things (food, toiletries, books, etc.) will add up to big expenses over time.

Also, try to hold off on starting a family. Children are a big obstacle to obtaining an education, especially when you are in your teenage years. Sooner or later, through personal responsibility or the courts, you will have to provide for your child. This will make it twice as hard to attend any educational institution and will also take time away from studying, even during online courses. It is very difficult to try to focus on curriculum if you have a small child in your life. Apart from that, your source of income (from which you will be supporting this child) will take a toll on the time you are able to devote to your work. Your libido is very high at this age, but you must resist and consider the consequences of your actions. Having a child early in life, especially when you have goals yet to be achieved, can be like obtaining a federal student loan because it will always be there, and you will always be responsible for it. Again, I was one of the lucky ones. I didn't always practice safe sex, and I was able to skate through my teenage years unscathed by the sentence of teen pregnancy.

I am not excusing the responsibility of the parents. It is of utmost importance that the parents share responsibility in teaching their children the difference between right and wrong. No parents want to see their children robbed of the opportunities that lie ahead in taking advantage of our educational system. But in the short and long of it, it is your child who will make his or her own decision for his or her future, and we can only point them in the right direction.

Precollege

When considering a college, you have to consider what you're going for. If you are going for computer science, engineering, or business, you may want to consider the school's reputation, the name, and quality. In qualifying a school to become a health-care professional, you must first consider whether it is recognized by the state licensing board. Most employers want to know if you are licensed and competent to perform your duties. The name and reputation of the school is a little less significant. I've worked with people who graduated from Ivy League schools, as well as those who have their online degrees, and I have seen very little difference in their competencies.

When you are looking for an education in health care, the cost to attend the institution is one of the more important things to think about. There are a variety of health-care programs available in the United States. Large and small colleges offer nursing and allied health courses of study. Seek out the type of school you want to attend—online, community college, a hospital certificate program, or a four-year college. What type of money do you want to spend? And what are your intentions for future employment? In 2014, the average cost of attending a community college can range anywhere between (before grants and scholarships) $1,000 per semester and $6,000 per semester. More than likely, the more competitive the college, the more it will cost. It's important to know the type of occupation you plan to attain because the further you go with your education, the more significant the type of school you attend becomes. For instance, if you intend on becoming a registered nurse and are only seeking to get your license, then an online school or community college is your best choice. The advantages are that online schools usually have no waiting lists, but they can be very expensive. And with community college, it's just the opposite; they are the least expensive but usually have long waiting lists of two years or more for the health-care professions in demand such as nursing, as well as many of the allied medical programs. If you're planning to go into management or obtaining postgraduate degrees such as your master's or PhD, you probably want to consider starting at a community college and not an online school. Although you can attend a four-year college with an online education, most community college credits transfer much easier than online credits, so you must have your licensure when you have an online degree. In any case, you should always strive to maintain the highest GPA possible. But that is much more important if you plan on obtaining a postgraduate degree. Because of the demand for postgraduate health-care professionals, most programs are highly competitive. Also the name and reputation of the schools you have attended may be significant, especially if you plan on climbing the corporate ladder toward becoming vice president or CEO of a large corporation.

You must also consider the type of occupation you are seeking because of the cost of your education. You have to make sure your investment will be enough so that when you graduate, there is a good chance you'll find a job and will be able to pay back the money that you borrowed in a short amount of time. If you spend $100,000 and you become a social worker, especially with a master's in social work, and your starting salary is only $55,000 a year or less, you will spend a much longer time paying this debt once you've obtained employment. On the contrary, if you spend this amount of money to become a nurse anesthetist and you're starting at $150,000 to $200,000 a year, then it probably won't take you as long to repay your debt. I am a huge Dave Ramsey fan, and I constantly hear how people spend hundreds of thousands of dollars and either can't find work or don't command the salaries commensurate with the debt they have accumulated—sad but true. It is very important to plan your education around your debt and not the other way around.

How Will I Pay My Room and Way?

Apply for as many grants and scholarships that are available to you, and get as much free money as you can. This is obviously the best scenario for attaining educational assistance. But it is also very competitive, and your GPA, among other things, must be competitive amid numerous applicants. Since most people don't have liquid cash to pay for their education, we rely on grants, loans, scholarships, and mostly federal student aid because it is the easiest for most Americans to obtain. There are a variety of loans available, including Stafford loans, Perkins, PLUS, and nonfederal loans, such as institutional, private, and state loans. The interest rates on these loans vary and must be taken into consideration during your application. Each loan has its own requirements and rules for qualification. In this day and age, it is almost a foregone conclusion in the minds of many that you must borrow money to obtain your education. But there are other paths as well.

Although there are a variety of grants and scholarships available, federal student loans are much easier to obtain and have fewer requirements. These loans are designed to cover most of your tuition, but when they become due, the lenders are unscrupulous in obtaining their money. They often employ the practice of garnishing your wages and repossessing your tax returns if your loans are not paid back in a timely manner. Unfortunately, because of the skyrocketing tuition rates, people feel they have no other choice but to borrow large amounts of money in the hope that they can pay these debts upon graduation and employment. But as we know, that is not always the case. Fortunately, there are routes you can take to avoid borrowing large amounts of money. Following these pathways requires patience and diligence. These are not always the most desired ways of reaching your goal, but you are much less likely to graduate from college in debt. Some alternatives include:

1) **Pay on time.** Take one class at a time. This gives you more time to focus on each subject. You will not be overwhelmed by taking multiple courses and can devote more of your time to each class. Spreading out the cost by taking one or two classes per semester can be much easier on the pocketbook as well. It may take a little longer, but it will be well worth it in the long run.

2) **Job tuition reimbursement.** Search for a job in the health-care industry. There are many positions that don't require formal training or certifications, such as home-health aides, medical assistants, medical secretaries, security guards, cafeteria attendants, environmental specialists, etc. Most health-care institutions offer tuition reimbursement for their employees if they remain at that institution for at least a year. Most require that you maintain a specific grade point average, and they have their own requirements for your working

status, whether full or part time. You may have to plan your classes according to your work schedule; some institutions are more flexible than others but will often work with you so you can complete your studies. You may have to alter your schedule as well. I know people who took night positions so they could study during the day. Of course, that is not always possible, so you must do what best fits your needs.

3) **Obtain training/certification.** There are many short-term, low-cost training programs that you can obtain to get your foot in the door at a health-care facility. There are a variety of courses available in low-level technical areas such as dialysis technician, phlebotomy, and certified nursing assistant. These positions will not only be useful in obtaining employment but will give you the training needed for higher-level positions in the future.

4) **Find employment with a school or university.** If you can secure employment at a college or university, they often offer free classes for the employee and the employee's family. Again, you may have to alter your work schedule or take classes around your work schedule. Depending on your diligence, it is possible to finish your studies at the normal rate of completion (two to four years). Another option is work-study, which provides part-time jobs for undergraduate and graduate students. These programs often encourage community service work and work related to the student's course of study.

5) **Borrow from family.** You should always consider this option last because you will still owe debt, and it

can also cause rifts in your relationships within the family if you do not pay them in a timely manner. Be sure to write a formal agreement of repayment and stick to that agreement.

6) **Keep one credit card.** You should obtain a credit card that is accepted by most merchants. I know you've probably heard many horror stories about the misuse of credit cards by irresponsible cardholders. Make sure your parents are aware or that you at least hold down a part-time job before you get one. Make sure the credit limit is not above $500 and try to pay the full balance every month. Keep this card in case you don't have cash on you or for emergencies. Do not use it as a regular way of paying your tuition. Use it just for partial payments or if the school does not accept payment on time.

And always remember to live within or below your means. Try to keep expenses low, according to your budget. As Dave Ramsey says, "Live like no one else today, so you can live like no one else tomorrow."

Bridge Programs

After you get your foot in the door and have gained about six months to a year of experience, you might want to look into a bridge program. A bridge program is a formal partnership between two postsecondary institutions that provides students with advanced standing in a degree program at one institution as recognition of previous academic experience in a similar field of study at another institution. Typically, a bridge program student holds a two-year degree and is seeking advancement in his or her profession by obtaining a four-year or graduate degree. There are also online bridge programs for CNAs to become LPNs; you might want to check with your state boards to make sure they are recognized. These programs are designed so that you can use the skills you've obtained to make a smooth transition to a higher-level patient care professional.

The cost of each program varies from institution to institution and program to program, so research each and make sure you choose the one that fits your needs. Most of these programs are relatively short—usually less than eighteen months—and very affordable, depending on which one you choose. The best thing about these programs is that there is no waiting list. You can apply to these programs and begin your studies right away. On completion, your hourly rate will most likely increase by five dollars or more.

These courses usually require only a high school diploma or GED. Although hospitals are not hiring LPNs or CNAs much anymore, opportunities still exist in a variety of settings, such as dialysis, assisted living, skilled nursing homes, and doctors' offices. These types of programs can accelerate the time it will take in achieving your ultimate goal in health care.

Licensure

Finally, you've graduated. You kept your expenses low, followed the path of least resistance, and have attained the right to sit for your licensure. I've always found that studying for the licensure is more effective when utilizing a fixed program of study, such as Kaplan NCLEX-RN review courses. You want to get the most up-to-date questions as possible, so don't borrow a book used years ago by someone who went through the program before you or borrow or buy used books from the library or bookstores; they are usually overpriced and not as up to date as the information you'll find taking a class. What worked best for me was actually taking a class and group study sessions. Not everyone needs to take such measures, but I find it much more helpful getting input from a group because of the camaraderie, focus, and the amount of information you can gather.

These types of courses will often utilize one of the nursing faculty and an optional amount of class time with the teacher who will walk through critical information and reasoning strategies you need to succeed. You'll get to go over multiple exam questions in the format similar to the actual licensure test, along with online resources. Get a leg up any way you can so that you can do well the first time. I had to take the test four times before I got a passing score, and let me tell you, it's very frustrating. I attribute my failures to my study habits. The one thing you can't do is give up. I know of nurses who failed their test numerous times and gave up. You'll never be satisfied with the money you're making, knowing you're only one test away from pulling down some real dollars. I understand the frustration involved, but in my opinion, the investment and time you put toward attaining your degree warrants extra due diligence in passing this test; in other words, never give up, no matter how many times you fail.

Location

Within the health-care field, there is a large demand for health-care professionals, and you have a choice of where you want to start your career. Wages vary from state to state, according to the cost of living. Nursing in California can average $85,000 to $90,000 per year, whereas a nurse in Alabama will make only $58,000 per year. Do you have family members in other states who might accommodate you temporarily? Are there other facilities or similar companies in the area that need health-care professionals? These are all important things to think about when you're considering how much control you want to have in your job and how to maximize the full potential of your wages. Typically, you will make less living in the Southeast than you will in the West. In states such as California, if you work over eight hours, you'll receive time and a half, and over twelve hours, you'll receive double time. There are websites you can go to that will give you a listing of the average salaries in each state.

When choosing a state, take into consideration the cost of living. If you're making $90,000 per year but your apartment is costing $3,000 a month, then your take-home pay may not reflect what you might expect.

If the cost of living is high, that means taxes are, too. If you are flexible and don't have many obligations, such as children, a mortgage, etc., then you have more choices that will enable you to go to the places where the money is. Keep in mind, though, that you want to continue to live within your means. Are you willing to travel? This is another way in which you can maximize your dollars by living in a low-cost state and traveling to a high-cost state temporarily. This also depends on your flexibility and willingness to temporarily, or permanently, leave your hometown. I will talk about travel agencies later on in the book. Do you have relatives with whom you may be able to stay temporarily in other states? I've seen nurses who were able to stay with close relatives temporarily for half of what it would cost to rent an apartment. You could save anywhere from $500 to $1,000 a month on each assignment, and if possible, extend your stay as long as it is acceptable to the renters/relatives.

As you work more and more in this field, think of some creative methods to save yourself a buck. Whether it's staying with family or friends, finding cheap housing, or moving temporarily to a high-paying state, there are multiple ways you can add to your bottom line.

Job Search

Are you ready to start searching for your new job? Hopefully, by the time you graduate, the job market will be as health-care friendly as it is currently. The US Department of Labor predicts faster than average growth for health-care professionals in the next decade. The most effective way, in my opinion, to secure a position in the shortest amount of time is to have personal or professional contacts or people you know who are already employed there. Not only will you stand a better chance of talking to the hiring manager, but you may have, through your contact, access to the company's intranet, which can provide you with information about the company and job openings you may not be able to get through an external search engine. You can use this information to better prepare yourself for the interview process, and you can research upcoming job openings that are not yet externally posted. This can save the time and money you'd expend going through an employment agency or headhunter group.

Alternatively, if you don't have contacts, you can use search engines and employment agencies and send out résumés to find that desired position. Sooner or later, you'll find a job. One technique that I have found very effective is an impromptu visit directly to the hiring manager. This can be very risky because you do not want to offend this person with an uninvited stopover. It depends on how desperate they are and how well their human resources department is performing in finding qualified candidates. If possible, talk to one of the employees on the floor and find out the hiring manager's schedule, which will give you a good indication of when to make that visit. If you find it is impossible, then just leave your résumé with that person on the floor. In either case, if done correctly, you will leave a lasting impression and increase your chances for securing employment at the facility.

To maximize your value in the interview process, be professional, look professional, and be prepared. Show that you've done your research and are ready to add value to your team and profits to the company's bottom line. Point out specific skills you possess that will promote quality and expertise. Remember, the facilities in this era are run by corporations; it is a business, and businesses want to make money. There is a fine line between giving quality care and making a profit, and you, as a health-care professional, must walk that tightrope very carefully. Don't be afraid to negotiate your salary. As well as the company being satisfied with you, you have to be satisfied with your earnings. Make sure you give them a salary range that is commensurate within the average wage in that state, but if you think you bring a little more to the table with your superior skills, then highlight those skills and be bold enough to explain why you deserve a higher than average salary or hourly wage. It is a risk but a risk worth taking.

Once you secure the job, make yourself invaluable at your facility. Be flexible and willing to learn every aspect of your job, your manager's job, and the technician's duties. I am a dialysis nurse, so I am responsible for administrating medications, performing patient assessments, and supervising the dialysis technicians, but I can also perform the dialysis technician's duties if he or she fails to show up for work or cannot perform as required. I am also able to run a dialysis facility by virtue of having a nursing license, without having a supervising manager present.

Maximize your worth by becoming an indispensable part of that team. Not only will you gain respect among your team members, but you will gain leverage to use upon your yearly evaluation, so you can maximize your wage increase.

Take advantage of your 401(k)/403(b). Contribute as much as you can each month and save as much money as you can from being taxed by the government. That includes using your health savings account (HSA) and the many perks offered at each facility, such as employee parking, corporate and local discounts, cafeteria privileges, and mileage reimbursement.

Beware of sign-on bonuses. They often look very attractive in advertisements. These tactics are used by companies to lure unsuspecting candidates or those in need of quick dollars to lock them into an agreement that will obligate them to stay with a company for a specific amount of time. What they don't say is that the money will be heavily taxed, and you may only get part of it at the beginning and the other part at the end. It may also take weeks to months after you have been employed to receive it. Also, along with that promise of quick money, the hiring manager may make promises to enhance this offer but inevitably rescinds some or all of the promises, for whatever reason, and you will still be obligated to finish your term or pay the money back in full.

After you get at least a year's worth of experience, you may want to look into changing your working status. At this point, you may be able to qualify for a wage differential that can add anywhere from two to five dollars per hour to your wages, and if you travel, they may offer mileage, that for me, personally, added $600 to $800 per month; every bit counts.

Since the signing of the new health-care act by President Obama, more and more health-care professionals have been emboldened to seek independence from the corporations, changing their work status to PRN/per diem to take more control over their schedules and to take advantage of the shift differentials it offers. In the past, most people were forced to work full time to get the full discount on their benefits package and health care. But now, with the onset of the new rules that prohibit insurance companies from excluding groups of people from qualifying for independent health-care insurance, it has become much more available. I have been able to work for numerous companies as a temporary worker without the threat of losing my health benefits just because I did not want to give all of my time to one entity. It is truly liberating. Because you have options, you can use this leverage to negotiate higher wages.

Another tip you can use to enhance your qualifications is to seek certification in your specialty. In dialysis, we can hold the designation of a certified nephrology nurse (CNN), and along with this, you can apply for an advanced cardiovascular life support certification (ACLS), which will highlight your years of service and expertise in the field. It will also expand your opportunities by making you more attractive to hiring managers, as well as possibilities of earning a higher wage. Seek out the certifications you qualify for in your chosen specialty and take full advantage of them.

Surprisingly, people don't often think about this, especially in health care, but staying healthy is a vital part of maximizing earning power. Not only must you be a role model to those you are caring for, but your body is your business, and without this, you cannot perform your job. Utilize the discounts provided by your benefits package and get your yearly checkup at the doctor's office. Stay ahead of the game, and prevent illnesses that may require emergency services and hospital stays. Exercise on a regular basis, and eat healthy foods to extend your life and earning power. A healthy body performs much better for a much longer period of time. You can also sell your sick time for cash instead of accumulating huge stores of it and losing a portion of it every year. I would also suggest using a portion of your personal time off (PTO) to give yourself the time needed (at least quarterly) to mend and maintain your mind, body, and spirit, as well as spending more time with your family.

Travel Agencies

Most travel agencies require at least two years of experience or more. Working with a travel agency is probably one of the best experiences I've had since joining the nursing profession. My first assignment was in California. I went to a remote part of Northern California near the Oregon border. I'm a city boy and was dreading three months in what looked to be a small, sleepy, boring town. On the contrary, it was just what I needed. The temperature never went above sixty or below fifty degrees, and it was either damp or rainy with occasional sunny days here and there. I was placed in a very neat and clean apartment close to the facility. The beach was about ten minutes away. I met some really nice people and actually came to love the sleepy town. From then on, I lost my fear of taking assignments at locations unknown to me. I've taken multiple travel assignments and enjoyed every minute of them.

For those who don't know what travel nursing entails, it's an industry that supplies nurses who travel to work temporarily in different parts of the state or country. The opportunity to travel is open to many allied health-care professionals, as well. Whether you are looking for personal adventure, professional growth, or feel the need to get away, it is a must that you take advantage of the opportunity. You can also travel outside of the United States, which may come with an offer for permanent employment. As of this writing, you can make anywhere between thirty and fifty dollars per hour. A typical travel agency will provide housing, tax-free stipends, health-care insurance, 401(k) with matching funds, licensure reimbursement, referral bonuses, and loyalty rewards. Some of the more established agencies may offer sick and vacation time, too.

The biggest advantage in working with a travel agency is the freedom of working for yourself. Although you are still considered an employee, after the completion of your assignment, you are free to explore other opportunities and gain new experiences without the dread of uncertainty you feel when leaving a full-time job. Another advantage, which I mentioned earlier, is the possibility of taking advantage of low-cost housing, such as renting a room or living with relatives, which can put more money into your pocket. There are also some agencies that accept contract workers where you are designated as self-employed. This allows you to pay your own taxes, which can save you money in tax deductions at the end of the year.

Some of the larger corporations may offer in-house travel that will allow you to travel to different locations around the country with your full-time job. The wages are slightly higher, and obviously you will keep your benefits package when your assignments are completed. Since the facilities you are working with are within the same company, another advantage is that you will be familiar with the policies and procedures, and that will make for a much smoother transition. The disadvantage is that you have no leverage to negotiate your wages, and you cannot entertain multiple offers, which can limit your opportunities to increase your wage.

Self-Employment

Many health-care professionals, such as nurses and physicians, have tried their hand at independent contracting and/or starting their own staffing agency. Both have similar regulatory limits, but when you own your own agency, you can hire your own employees rather than just subcontracting other professionals. Either way, your business has the potential for earnings far surpassing that of an average employee. You can set your own hours, use your own equipment, follow your own policies and procedures, and enjoy all the perks of owning your own business, including decreased tax liabilities. Unfortunately for independent contractors, because of recent negative IRS rulings, it has become much more risky to adopt this practice. The IRS may not view you as self-employed in a health-care facility setting due to using the facility's equipment, working scheduled hours, and functioning under that facility's policies and procedures, which could open the payor up to being liable for back taxes. Furthermore, Medicare and Medicaid may pull funding from facilities using independent contractors for patient care, and the likelihood of getting audited as an independent contractor is very high. Back taxes, penalties, and interest can be devastating for the payer. You must think long and hard before delving into this type of occupation, and you must be prepared to legally defend your contract.

Home care, although becoming increasingly scrutinized by the IRS, is a much safer specialty because you can use private payers, excluding Medicare and Medicaid. Your contract with the payer must be indisputable and legally ironclad. If you are well educated and prepared, this venture can pay off big, but you must measure the pros and cons of this gamble and judge for yourself if it is worth your efforts and time.

Most ventures come with risks and rewards. The health-care industry is no different. In the end it is one of the few ways to start from nothing to forming a foundation toward changing your lifestyle and having the ability to support your family and possibly changing your family tree. With good planning, patience, and a deep desire to accomplish your goal, anything is possible. Everyone can do it regardless of their socioeconomic status or upbringing. The opportunities are there for the taking. Grasp them and let them take you to greatness!

Conclusion

I consider myself lucky to have built my career in the health-care field. It is one of the few occupations that offers almost guaranteed employment after graduation. But just like any other career, you can find yourself a slave to your job through debt, and it doesn't matter how much money you make. Unless you make good decisions in the initial phase of your career, it may be difficult to reap the benefits that come with investing in a good education. In today's economic climate, it is very easy to be sent into the jaws of long-term debt. Fortunately, because of the need for health-care professionals, this field can be an oasis from impending drought, and many, like myself, have been able to take advantage of this opportunity. I had to run the gauntlet of trial and error before realizing the correct path to prosperity and financial freedom. It can be a long road if you do not follow the correct path the first time. Research, study, and follow the people who have already been down that road, and you may have a much more pleasant experience. I hope this book has given you a clear view on which path to follow. Good luck to you all!

Acknowledgements

This book is dedicated to my son Charles. You are the inspiration for all I do.

I would also like to give thanks to mom and dad for all of your support.

I would also like to thank Aisha Scott and Tony Gordon for giving me the inspiration to write this book.